RENAL DIET COOKBOOK FOR BEGINNERS 2024

A Delightful Exploration into Health with 50 Recipes That Are Safe for Kidneys

David Gomer

Table of Content

INTRODUCTION

Welcome to the "Renal Delights Cookbook," your one-stop shop for tasty and kidney-friendly dishes that will help you maintain a healthy renal diet. As we embark on this gastronomic adventure, it's critical to understand the importance of living a renal-friendly lifestyle and the role diet plays in kidney health.

Living with kidney disease necessitates paying close attention to dietary choices, highlighting the need to manage minerals such as potassium, phosphorus, and sodium. This cookbook seeks to provide you with the information and culinary skills necessary to prepare meals that not only satisfy your taste buds but also contribute to the general health of your kidneys.

In this introduction, we'll look at the basics of renal diets and explain why some dietary changes are so important for those with kidney disease. We'll also discuss the significance of nutrient control and how these dishes adhere to the concepts of a renal-friendly lifestyle.

Renal Diets Explained

Renal diets are specifically designed to fulfill the dietary demands of those who have kidney problems. These diets concentrate on controlling the intake of specific nutrients that can affect kidney function, such as potassium, phosphorus, and sodium. Individuals can better maintain their renal health and slow the progression of kidney-related disorders by carefully regulating these factors.

The Importance of Nutrient Management

Maintaining a delicate nutritional balance is critical for those suffering from kidney problems. High potassium, phosphorus, and salt levels can put a load on the kidneys, potentially leading to difficulties. The dishes in this cookbook are meticulously developed, taking into account the recommended guidelines for these nutrients, resulting in a harmonious balance that promotes renal health without sacrificing flavor.

As we turn the pages of the "Renal Delights Cookbook," you'll find a wide range of dishes for breakfast, lunch, dinner, snacks, and even desserts. Each recipe has been carefully selected to be not just kidney-friendly but also delicious. These ideas range from inventive breakfast bowls to tasty dinner wonders and refreshing beverages, and are intended to make your renal diet both pleasurable and nourishing.

This cookbook aspires to be a trusted friend in your kitchen, whether you're navigating a renal diet for yourself or helping a loved one on this path. Each recipe includes detailed instructions, nutritional information, and recommendations to help you make smart meal choices. Our mission is to inspire and enable you to enjoy the pleasures of good food while putting kidney health first.

The next chapters contain a thorough collection of 50 recipes, each of which contributes to a varied and savory renal diet. So join me on this gastronomic trip where taste meets kidney health and every bite is a step toward wellbeing. Welcome to the "Renal Delights Cookbook," where nourishment and flavor join together to assist your kidney health journey.

The Fundamentals of Renal-Friendly Ingredients

Starting a renal-friendly diet entails more than just choosing recipes; it necessitates a thorough grasp of the elements that serve as the foundation of these nutritious and kidney-conscious meals. This part will go over the fundamentals of renal-friendly ingredients, with a focus on low-potassium diets, good phosphorus management, and the significance of sodium restriction.

Foods Low in Potassium

Potassium is an essential mineral that aids in a variety of body activities, including neuron and muscle cell communication. Excess potassium, on the other hand, can be difficult to process in people with impaired kidney function. This portion of the cookbook focuses on including low-potassium foods such as berries, apples, cucumbers, and green beans. These options provide a balance that promotes renal health while maintaining the diversity and vibrancy of your meals.

Phosphorus Control

Another mineral that must be carefully considered in renal diets is phosphorus. While needed for bone health and energy production, high phosphorus levels might be troublesome for people who have kidney problems. The dishes in this cookbook include an emphasis on phosphorus-conscious ingredients. Cauliflower, quinoa, and egg whites are examples of foods that not only supply essential nutrients but also adhere to the principles of good phosphorus management.

Restriction on Sodium

Sodium, which is mostly found in salt, is a mineral that can cause fluid retention and raise blood pressure. Sodium limitation is critical for patients with renal problems to maintain optimal kidney function. The cookbook provides a variety of herbs, spices, and alternative seasonings to enhance flavor without overuse of salt. You can enjoy delicious meals while sticking to sodium restrictions that support overall kidney health by integrating these options.

Making knowledgeable grocery store decisions is necessary for navigating the world of renal-friendly ingredients. This portion of the cookbook teaches you how to read labels and detect hidden sources of potassium, phosphorus, and sodium. With this knowledge, you may confidently choose items that correspond to your dietary needs, ensuring that each component of your meal contributes to your renal health.

This section provides practical meal planning recommendations in addition to showcasing specific low-potassium, phosphorus-conscious, and low-sodium foods. It delves into the art of preparing well-balanced meals that not only meet nutritional requirements but also excite your taste buds. Whether you're a rookie or a seasoned home cook, these renal-friendly ingredient insights can help you make informed decisions and transform your kitchen into a zone where health and flavor dwell happily.

Understanding and appreciating the fundamentals of renal-friendly ingredients lays the groundwork for creating meals that nourish both your body and your taste buds. So, let's go grocery shopping with confidence, knowing that every product we choose adds to a renal-friendly lifestyle that promotes optimal kidney health.

CHAPTER 1

Breakfast Favorites

Breakfast Bowl with Quinoa

Composition:

• 1 cup quinoa, cooked

• 1/2 cup fresh berries

• A cup of chopped nuts, preferably walnuts or almonds

• 1 tablespoon honey

• 1/2 cup Greek yogurt (low-fat)

Directions:

1. Combine the cooked quinoa and Greek yogurt in a mixing basin.

2. Drizzle with honey and top with fresh berries and chopped almonds.

3. Mix together and serve this protein- and nutrient-rich breakfast bowl.

Nutritional Facts:

• 350 calories

• 15g protein

• 55g carbohydrate

• 7g fiber

• 8g of good fats

Oatmeal with Apples and Cinnamon

Composition:

• 1/2 cup oats, old-fashioned

• 1 cup almond milk, unsweetened

• 1 medium-sized diced apple

• 1/2 teaspoon cinnamon powder

• 1 tbsp. chopped almonds

Directions:

1. Combine oats and almond milk in a saucepan. Cook until the oats are soft over medium heat.

2. Mix in the diced apples and cinnamon.

3. When done, transfer to a bowl and top with chopped almonds.

• Nutritional Facts:

• 300 calories

• 8g protein

• 50g carbohydrates

• 10g fiber

• 6g of good fats

Omelet with Vegetables and Egg Whites

Composition:

- three egg whites

- 1/4 cup chopped red and green bell peppers

- 1/4 cup chopped tomatoes

- 1/4 cup spinach, chopped

- 1 tsp feta cheese (optional)

- Then add salt and pepper

Directions:

1. Season the egg whites with salt and pepper.

2. Sauté bell peppers, tomatoes, and spinach in a nonstick skillet until soft.

3. Pour the egg whites over the vegetables and heat until set. If preferred, top with feta cheese.

Nutritional Facts:

- 180 calories

- 20g protein

- 8g carbohydrate

- 2g fiber

- 7g of good fats

Pancakes with Blueberries and Buckwheat Flour

Composition:

- half a cup of buckwheat flour

- Half a cup of almond flour

- 1 tsp baking powder

- Half a cup of almond milk

- 1/2 cup blueberries, fresh

- 1 tsp maple syrup (optional)

Directions:

1. Buckwheat flour, almond flour, and baking powder should be combined in a mixing dish.

2. To make a batter, gradually add the almond milk. Fold in the blueberries gently.

3. Griddle spoonfuls of batter till golden brown. If desired, drizzle with maple syrup.

Nutritional Facts:

- 250 calories

- 9g protein

- 35g carbohydrate

- 6g fiber

• 8g of good fats

Parfait with Greek Yogurt

Composition

• 1 cup Greek yogurt (low-fat)

• 1/2 cup low-sugar granola

• 1/2 cup berries of your choice (strawberries, blueberries, or raspberries)

• 1 teaspoon honey

Directions:

1. Layer Greek yogurt, granola, and mixed berries in a glass.

2. Layer again, concluding with a sprinkle of honey on top.

Nutritional Facts:

- 320 calories

- 15g protein

- 45g carbohydrate

- 7g fiber

- 9g of good fats

Tips:

- Tailor these recipes to your nutritional needs and preferences.

- For added variation, try different fruits, nuts, and seeds.

- Maintain portion management and seek tailored dietary advice from a healthcare practitioner.

Start your day off right with these kidney-friendly breakfast treats. These dishes not only meet the needs of your kidneys, but they also add a blast of taste to your morning routine. Remember that a nutritious breakfast sets the tone for the rest of the day, and with these recipes, you can prioritize both taste and renal health.

CHAPTER 2

Lunch Concoctions

Salad of Grilled Chicken with Lemon Vinaigrette

Composition:

- 4 ounces sliced grilled chicken breast

- 2 cups salad greens, mixed

- 1/2 cup halved cherry tomatoes

- 1/4 cup chopped cucumber

- 1/4 cup finely chopped red onion

• 1 tsp feta cheese (optional)

• 1 tablespoon olive oil, 1 tablespoon lemon juice, salt, and pepper

Directions:

1. On a platter, layer salad greens, grilled chicken, cherry tomatoes, cucumber, and red onion.

2. If preferred, top the salad with feta cheese.

3. Combine the olive oil, lemon juice, salt, and pepper in a mixing bowl. Drizzle the dressing over the salad.

Nutritional Facts:

• 400 calories

• 30g protein

• 15g carbohydrate

- 4g fiber

- 22g of healthy fats

Soup with Lentils and Vegetables

Composition

- 1 cup green lentils, dry

- 4 cups veggie broth

- 1 cup sliced carrots

- 1 cup chopped celery

- 1 cup chopped zucchini

- 1 cup chopped spinach

- 1 tablespoon cumin

- Then add salt and pepper

Directions:

1. In a pot, add lentils and vegetable broth. Bring the water to a boil.

2. Mix in the carrots, celery, zucchini, and cumin. Cook until the lentils and veggies are soft.

3. Stir in the spinach. Add salt and pepper according to your taste.

Nutritional Facts:

- 350 calories

- 18g protein

- 60g carbohydrates

- 15g fiber

- 2g of healthy fat

Wrap with turkey and avocado

Composition:

- 4 ounces lean turkey slices

- 1 whole-wheat wrap

- 1 tablespoon hummus

- 1/2 sliced avocado

- 1/2 cup mixed greens (arugula, spinach, etc.)

- 1 tbsp (optional) Greek yogurt

Directions:

1. Layer the wrap with hummus, turkey slices, avocado, and mixed greens.

2. Drizzle Greek yogurt over the filling if desired.

3. Wrap the wrap securely and cut it in half.

Nutritional Facts:

- 420 calories

- 25g protein

- 35g carbohydrate

- 8g fiber

- 20g of healthy fats

Stuffed peppers with quinoa and shrimp

Composition:

- 1/2 cup cooked quinoa

- 8 large bell peppers, peeled and halved

- 1 pound peeled and deveined shrimp

- 1 cup chopped tomatoes

- 1/2 cup rinsed and drained black beans

- 1/4 cup chopped fresh cilantro

- 1 tablespoon cumin

- 1/2 tsp smoked paprika

• Then add salt and pepper

Directions:

1. Ensure to heat the oven to 375 degrees Fahrenheit (190 degrees Celsius).

2. Combine cooked quinoa, shrimp, chopped tomatoes, black beans, cilantro, cumin, smoked paprika, salt, and pepper in a mixing bowl.

3. Fill each half of a bell pepper with the quinoa-shrimp mixture. Bake until the peppers are soft.

Nutritional Facts:

• 380 calories

• 30g protein

• 35g carbohydrate

• 8g fiber

- 12g of healthy fats

Quiche with Spinach and Feta

Composition:

- 1 whole-grain pie crust (pre-made)

- four big eggs

- 1-quart skim milk

- 2 cups chopped fresh spinach

- 1/2 cup crumbled feta cheese

- 1/4 cup coarsely chopped red onion

- Then add salt and pepper

Directions:

1. Ensure to heat the oven to 375 degrees Fahrenheit (190 degrees Celsius).

2. Whisk together the eggs and milk in a mixing basin. Add the spinach, feta cheese, red onion, salt, and pepper to taste.

3. Fill the pie shell with the contents and bake until the quiche is set and gently browned.

Nutritional Facts:

• 320 calories

• 18g protein

• 20g carbohydrates

• 2g fiber

• 18g of healthy fats

Tips:

• Modify serving amounts according to individual dietary requirements.

• Include a variety of bright vegetables for extra nutrition.

• Drink water or herbal teas throughout the day to stay hydrated.

These lunch compositions are intended to give a filling and nutritious midday meal while keeping to renal-friendly guidelines. Enjoy the flavors and textures in these meals, and make them a regular part of your journey to better kidney health.

CHAPTER 3

Dinner Surprises

Salmon Baked with Dill Sauce

Composition:

- 6 ounces salmon filet

- 1 teaspoon olive oil

- 1 tsp. dried dill

- 1/2 tsp garlic powder

- Then add salt and pepper

- Dill Sauce: 2 tbsp Greek yogurt, 1 tsp fresh dill, 1 tsp lemon juice

Directions:

1.1. Bring the temperature of the oven up to 400 degrees Fahrenheit (200 degrees Celsius).

2. Salmon should be rubbed with olive oil, dried dill, garlic powder, salt, and pepper. Bake until the salmon is done.

3. For the dill sauce, combine Greek yogurt, fresh dill, and lemon juice. Serve with baked salmon.

Nutritional Facts:

• 400 calories

• 30g protein

• 2g Carbohydrates

• 0g fiber

• 28g of healthy fats

Risotto with Portobello Mushrooms

Composition:

- 1 pound Arborio rice

- 4 cups veggie broth

- 2 tbsp of olive oil

- 1/2 cup onion, diced

- 2 minced garlic cloves

- 4 sliced portobello mushrooms

- 1/2 cup white wine, dry

- 1/4 cup Parmesan cheese, grated

- Then add salt and pepper

Directions:

1. Heat olive oil in a saucepan and sauté onions and garlic until transparent.

2. Cook until the Arborio rice is lightly browned.

3. Add the white wine and sliced portobello mushrooms. Add vegetable broth gradually until the rice is done.

4. Finish with a sprinkle of Parmesan cheese, salt, and pepper.

Nutritional Facts:

• 380 calories

• 10g protein

• 55g carbohydrate

• 4g fiber

• 14g of healthy fats

Stir-fry with Chickpeas and Vegetables

Composition:

- 1 can (15 oz) washed and drained chickpeas

- 2 cups florets broccoli

- 1 sliced bell pepper

- 1 julienned carrot

- 2 tbsp of soy sauce

1 teaspoon sesame oil

- 1 teaspoon minced ginger

- 2 minced garlic cloves

Directions:

1. Sesame oil should be heated in a wok or skillet. Ginger and garlic should be sautéed until aromatic.

2. Combine chickpeas, broccoli, bell pepper, and carrot in a mixing bowl. Cook until the vegetables are soft.

3. Toss the stir-fry with the soy sauce to incorporate.

Nutritional Facts:

• 320 calories

• 14g protein

• 45g carbohydrate

• 12g fiber

• 10g of healthy fats

Chicken Breast with Roasted Herbs

Composition:

• 2 skinless, boneless chicken breasts

• 1 teaspoon olive oil

- 1 tsp dried herbs (rosemary, thyme, oregano)

- 1/2 tsp garlic powder

- Then add salt and pepper

Directions:

1. Ensure to heat the oven to 375 degrees Fahrenheit (190 degrees Celsius).

2. Rub olive oil, dried herbs, garlic powder, salt, and pepper on chicken breasts.

3. Roast until the chicken is thoroughly done and the juices run clear.

Nutritional Facts:

- 280 calories

- 30g protein

- 0g Carbohydrates

- 0g fiber

- 16g of healthy fats

Tomato Basil Sauce with Zucchini Noodles

Composition

- 2 medium spiralized zucchinis

- 1 cup halved cherry tomatoes

- 1/4 cup chopped fresh basil

- 2 tbsp of olive oil

- 2 minced garlic cloves

- Then add salt and pepper

- Parmesan cheese, grated (optional)

Directions:

1. Heat olive oil in a pan and sauté garlic till golden.

2. Mix in the zucchini noodles and cherry tomatoes. Cook until the noodles are soft.

3. Add the fresh basil, salt, and pepper to taste. Sprinkle with Parmesan cheese, if desired.

Nutritional Facts:

• 220 calories

• 5g protein

• 15g carbohydrate

• 5g fiber

• 17g of healthy fats

Tips:

• Tailor the seasonings to your taste preferences.

• For a nutrient-dense dinner, include a range of colorful vegetables.

• Keep track of portion amounts to ensure they correspond to your nutritional requirements.

These dinnertime miracles are designed with both flavor and renal health in mind. As you continue on your journey to support optimal kidney health via thoughtful and delicious eating, enjoy these nutritious and fulfilling dishes.

CHAPTER 4

Side Dish Extravaganza

Cauliflower Mash

Composition:

• 1 medium cauliflower head, sliced into florets

• 2 minced garlic cloves

• 2 tbsp of olive oil

• Then add salt and pepper

• Garnish with fresh chives

Directions:

1. Cauliflower should be steamed or boiled until soft.

2. Cauliflower should be mashed with minced garlic, olive oil, salt, and pepper.

3. Garnish with chopped fresh chives.

Nutritional Facts:

• 120 calories

• 5g protein

• 12g Carbohydrates

• 6g fiber

• 7g of good fats

Brussels Sprouts, Roasted

Composition:

• 1 pound trimmed and halved Brussels sprouts

• 2 tbsp of olive oil

• 1 tsp balsamic vinegar

• Then add salt and pepper

• 2 tbsp. grated Parmesan cheese

Directions:

1. Toss Brussels sprouts with olive oil, balsamic vinegar, salt, and pepper in a mixing bowl.

2. Cook till golden brown in the oven.

3. Before serving, top with Parmesan cheese.

Nutritional Facts:

• 160 calories

• 8g protein

- 18g carbohydrate

- 8g fiber

- 8g of good fats

Brown Rice with Lemon Herb

Composition:

- 1 cup cooked brown rice

- 1 lemon's zest and juice

- 1 tablespoon chopped fresh parsley

- 1 tablespoon chopped fresh dill

- Then add salt and pepper

Directions:

1. Combine cooked brown rice, lemon zest, lemon juice, parsley, and dill in a mixing bowl.

2. Season with salt and pepper to taste.

Nutritional Facts:

• 200 calories

• 5g protein

• 40g carbohydrates

• 3g fiber

• 2g of healthy fat

Almondine, Green Beans

Composition:

• 1 pound trimmed green beans

• 2 tbsp. almonds, sliced

• 1 teaspoon olive oil

• 1 tbsp. lemon juice

• Then add salt and pepper to taste

Directions:

1. Green beans should be blanched in boiling water before being shocked in icy water.

2. Toast sliced almonds in a skillet until brown.

3. Toss green beans with olive oil, lemon juice, toasted almonds, salt, and pepper in a large mixing bowl.

Nutritional Facts:

• 180 calories

• 6g protein

• 15g carbohydrate

• 7g fiber

• 12g of healthy fats

Wedges of Sweet Potato

Composition:

• 2 medium sweet potatoes, peeled and cut into wedges

• 2 tbsp of olive oil

• 1 tsp smoked paprika

• Optional: 1/2 teaspoon cayenne pepper

• Then add salt and pepper

Directions:

1. A temperature of 400 degrees Fahrenheit (200 degrees Celsius) should be set for the oven.

2. Toss smoked paprika, cayenne pepper, salt, and pepper into sweet potato slices.

3. Cook until golden brown and crispy.

Nutritional Facts:

• 220 calories

• 3g protein

• 40g carbohydrates

• 6g fiber

• 7g of good fats

Tips:

• Tailor the seasoning amounts to your taste preferences.

• For an added taste boost, add fresh herbs.

• To get more fiber, choose whole-grain rice.

These amazing side dish ideas are designed to complement your main courses while maintaining a mix of flavors and kidney-friendly nutritional content. Enhance your meals with these delectable and nutritious accompaniments, each of which contributes to the pleasure and well-being of your eating experience.

CHAPTER 5

Snack Sensations

Bites of cucumber and hummus

- 1 cucumber, cut

- 1/2 cup hummus

- cherry tomatoes for garnish

- fresh parsley for garnish

Directions:

1. Place a dollop of hummus on top of each cucumber slice.

2. Garnish with fresh parsley and cherry tomatoes.

Nutritional Facts:

• 80 calories

• 4g protein

• 10g Carbohydrates

• 3g fiber

• 4g healthy fats

Smoothie with Mixed Berries

• 1 cup mixed berries (strawberries, blueberries, and raspberries)

- 1/2 cup low-fat Greek yogurt

- 1/2 cup almond milk

- 1 tbsp chia seeds

- 1 tsp honey (optional)

Directions:

1. In a blender, combine the mixed berries, Greek yogurt, almond milk, and chia seeds until smooth.

2. If desired, sweeten with honey.

Nutritional Facts:

- 150 calories

- 8g protein

20g carbohydrates

6g fiber

5g healthy fats

Nuts and Seeds Trail Mix

- 1/4 cup almonds

- 1/4 cup walnuts

- 1/4 cup pumpkin seeds

- 1/4 cup dried cranberries

- 1/4 cup dark chocolate chips (optional)

Directions:

1. Combine almonds, walnuts, pumpkin seeds, dried cranberries, and dark chocolate chips in a mixing bowl.

2. Divide into snack-sized portions.

Nutritional Facts:

- 200 caloriesProtein

6g Carbohydrates

15g Fiber:

4g Healthy Fats: 15g

Edamame Snack Pods

- 1 cup steamed edamame

- 1 teaspoon sesame oil

- 1/2 teaspoon sea salt

- 1/2 teaspoon sesame seeds

Directions:

1. Combine steamed edamame, sesame oil, sea salt, and sesame seeds in a mixing bowl.

2. Divide into snack-sized servings.

Nutritional Facts:

- 120 calories

- 11g protein

- 8g carbohydrates

- 4g fiber

- 5g of good fats

Pineapple and Cottage Cheese Salsa

Ingredients

1/2 cup low-fat cottage cheese

1/2 cup diced fresh pineapple

1/4 cup finely chopped red bell pepper

1 tablespoon minced fresh cilantro

1 teaspoon lime juice

Directions:

1. Combine cottage cheese, diced pineapple, red bell pepper, cilantro, and lime juice in a mixing bowl.

2. Plate or serve in individual portions.

Nutritional Facts:

• 130 calories

• 12g protein

• 18g carbohydrates

• 2g fiber

• 1g healthy fat

Tips:

• Adjust serving amounts to meet your dietary requirements.

• For a lower sugar level, choose unsweetened yogurt and milk.

• For trail mix, try different nut and seed combinations.

These snack sensations are not only delicious, but they are also intended to satisfy your appetites while keeping a kidney-friendly balance. Whether you're looking for a quick snack or something more substantial, these snacks provide a variety of textures and flavors that contribute to both enjoyment and optimal kidney health.

CHAPTER 6

Dessert Delights

Chia Seed Pudding

- 3 tablespoons chia seeds

- 1 cup almond milk

- 1/2 teaspoon vanilla extract

- 1 tablespoon maple syrup

- Fresh berries to serve as a garnish

Directions

1. In a container, combine chia seeds, almond milk, vanilla essence, and maple syrup.

2. Refrigerate the mixture overnight, or until it thickens.

3. Before serving, top with fresh berries.

Nutritional Facts:

• 180 calories

• 4g protein

25g carbohydrates

10g fiber

7g healthy fats

Cinnamon-Baked Apple

• 2 apples, cored and halved

• 1 teaspoon cinnamon

• 1 tablespoon honey

• 2 tablespoons chopped walnuts

Directions:

1. Ensure to heat the oven to 375 degrees Fahrenheit (190 degrees Celsius).

2. Arrange the apple halves on a baking pan. Drizzle with honey and sprinkle with cinnamon.

3. Bake until the apples are soft. Before serving, sprinkle with chopped walnuts.

Nutritional Facts:

• 160 calories

• 2g protein

35g carbohydrates

6g fiber

3g healthy fats

Frozen Banana Bites

Ingredients:

2 ripe bananas, sliced

• 1/4 cup peanut butter

- 1/4 cup melted dark chocolate

- Finely chopped nuts for coating

Directions:

1. Spread peanut butter on pieces of banana and sandwich them together.

2. Drizzle melted dark chocolate over each banana sandwich.

3. Roll in chopped nuts and place in the freezer until the chocolate solidifies.

Nutritional Facts:

- 220 calories

- 4g protein

28g carbohydrates

4g fiber

12g healthy fats

Greek Yogurt with Granola Parfait

Ingredients:

1 cup Greek yogurt (low-fat)

• 1/2 cup low-sugar granola

• 1/2 cup mixed berries (strawberries, blueberries, or raspberries)

• 1 tablespoon honey

Directions

1. Layer Greek yogurt, granola, and mixed berries in a glass.

2. Layer again, concluding with a drizzle of honey on top.

Nutritional Facts:

• 320 caloriesProtein

15g Carbohydrates

45g Fiber

7g Healthy Fats

Avocado Chocolate Mousse

Ingredients

2 ripe avocados

• 1/4 cup cocoa powder

• 1/4 cup maple syrup

• 1 teaspoon vanilla essence

• pinch of salt

Directions

1. In a food processor, combine avocados, cocoa powder, maple syrup, vanilla extract, and salt until smooth.

2. Place in the refrigerator before serving.

Nutritional Facts:

• 250 calories

• 3g protein

30g carbohydrates

10g fiber

15g healthy fats

Tips:

• Tailor the sweetness to your taste preferences.

• For added diversity, use seasonal fruits.

• Add nuts and seeds for added crunch and nutrition.

These dessert treats are designed to bring a delightful ending to your meals while maintaining kidney health. Enjoy the rich textures and aromas of these delicacies, which all contribute to a delicious dining experience that is in line with your nutritional goals.

CHAPTER 7

Beverages for Kidney Health

Maintaining optimal kidney health entails not just eating mindfully but also staying hydrated with beverages that promote renal function. Here are the ingredients, proportions, and nutritional values for five kidney-friendly beverages.

Cucumber Mint Infused Water

Ingredients:

1/2 sliced cucumber

• fresh mint leaves

• 4 cups water

* ice cubes

Directions:

1. In a pitcher, combine cucumber slices and fresh mint leaves.

2. Add water and chill for several hours to allow flavors to integrate.

3. Pour over ice for a pleasant and hydrating beverage.

Nutritional Facts:

* Calories: 0

* No protein, fat, or carbs

* Excellent hydration

Hibiscus Ginger Iced Tea

* 2 hibiscus tea bags (optional)

* 1 tablespoon sliced fresh ginger

• 4 cups boiling water

• 1 tablespoon honey (optional)

• Lemon slices for decoration

Directions:

1. Boil water with hibiscus tea bags and sliced ginger for 10 minutes.

2. If desired, sweeten with honey and set aside to cool.

3. For a delicious iced tea, serve over ice with lemon slices.

Nutritional Facts:

• 20 calories

• No protein, fat, or major carbohydrates

• Excellent hydration

Berry Blast Smoothie

• 1/2 cup mixed berries (strawberries, blueberries, raspberries)

• 1/2 cup low-fat Greek yogurt

• Half a cup of water or almond milk1 teaspoon chia seeds

• Cubes of ice

Directions:

1. Puree the mixed berries, Greek yogurt, water or almond milk, and chia seeds in a food processor until smooth.

2. For a refreshing and nutritious smoothie, add ice cubes.

Nutritional Facts:

• 150 caloriesProtein:

10g Carbohydrates:

20g Fiber:

6g Healthy Fats: 5g

Turmeric Golden Latte

1 cup unsweetened almond milk

- 1/2 teaspoon turmeric powder

- 1/4 teaspoon cinnamon

- 1/4 teaspoon ginger powder

- 1 tbsp honey (optional)

Directions:

1. In a saucepan, combine the almond milk, turmeric powder, cinnamon, and ginger powder.

2. If desired, sweeten with honey.

3. Pour into a mug and enjoy this anti-inflammatory and warming beverage.

Nutritional Facts:

• 40 calories

• 1g protein

8g carbohydrates

1g fiber

2g healthy fats

Watermelon Lime Cooler

Ingredients:

2 cups fresh watermelon, diced

2 limes' juice

1 tablespoon chopped fresh mint

2 cups cold water; ice cubes

Directions:

1. Puree the watermelon cubes, lime juice, and fresh mint in a food processor until smooth.

2. Remove the pulp from the mixture by straining it.

3. Combine with cold water and serve over ice for a refreshing and tasty drink.

Nutritional Facts:

- 60 calories

- 1g protein

15g carbohydrates

1g fiber

0g healthy fats

Tips:

• Adjust the sweetness level to suit your tastes.

• Be aware of portion proportions, especially while making smoothies.

• Include these beverages as part of a well-balanced, kidney-friendly diet.

These kidney-friendly beverages come in a variety of tastes and provide critical hydration as well as potential health benefits. These recipes cater to both your taste buds and your kidney health, whether you're searching for a refreshing infusion, a healthy smoothie, or a cozy warm drink. To support optimum kidney function, include these beverages in your regular regimen.

CHAPTER 8

Recipes for Special Occasion Use

When it comes to celebrating special occasions, one of the best ways to take pleasure in the moment is to do so by preparing meals that are both delicious and kidney-friendly. This article presents five recipes that are suitable for special occasions and not only taste amazing but also are in line with renal health. There is a list of ingredients, measurements, and nutritional values included in each dish.

Salmon prepared on the grill with a lemon-dill sauce

Ingredients

• 4 salmon filets, each weighing 6 ounces

• Olive oil, two tablespoons worth

A total of two teaspoons of chopped fresh dill

One lemon, with the zest and the juice

• Then add salt and pepper

Directions

a. 1. First, bring the grill up to a medium-high temperature.

2. The salmon filets should be seasoned with salt and pepper after being brushed with olive oil.

3. Cook on the grill for four to five minutes per side, or until the meat is completely cooked through.

4. To make the sauce, combine the chopped dill, lemon zest, and lemon juice. On top of the grilled fish, serve.

Nutritional facts

• The number of calories is 350

30 grams of protein

• Carbohydrates: 0.2 grams

• Fiber content: 0 grams

• 22 grams of healthy fats

Chicken Breast Stuffed with Spinach and Mushrooms Recipe

Ingredients

• Four chicken breasts that are skinless and boneless

a cup of mushrooms, cut as needed

A total of two cups of chopped fresh spinach

One-fourth of a cup of crumbled feta cheese

• Two large cloves of garlic, minced

Olive oil, one tablespoon's worth

• Then add salt and pepper

Directions

a. 1. Get the oven up to 375 F (190 C) before you start.

2. To wilt the mushrooms, spinach, and garlic, sauté them in olive oil in a pan until they are tender.

3. Each chicken breast should have a pocket cut into it, and the mushroom-spinach mixture should be stuffed into the pocket.

4. Cook the chicken in the oven until it is just done.

Nutritional Facts:

• The number of calories is 280

35 grams of protein

Four grams of carbohydrates

• Fiber content: 2 grams

• 12 grams of healthy fats

Peppers that are stuffed with quinoa and vegetables

Ingredients

• Four large bell peppers, separated from their seeds and cut in half

A cup of cooked quinoa, one cup

1 cup of black beans, drained and rinsed before serving

• One cup of kernels of corn

.A half cup of cherry tomatoes, sliced in half, is required.

• One-half cup of red onion, cut very finely

a single teaspoon of cumin

One-half of a teaspoon of chili powder

• Then add salt and pepper

Directions

1. Ensure to heat the oven to 375 degrees Fahrenheit (190 degrees Celsius).

2. Quinoa that has been cooked, black beans, corn, cherry tomatoes, red onion, cumin, chili powder, salt, and pepper should be combined in a bowl; mix well.

3. The quinoa-vegetable mixture should be stuffed into each half of the bell pepper. Roast the peppers until they are soft.

Nutritional Facts

• The number of calories is 320

• Protein: ten grams

Carbohydrates: sixty grams

12 grams of fiber

• 5 grams of healthy fats

The Parmesan of eggplant

Ingredients

• Two large eggplants, cut into chunks

• Two cups of low-sodium versions of marinara sauce

• One cup of shredded mozzarella cheese made from part skim,

• One-half cup of grated Parmesan goat cheese

a half cup of breadcrumbs made from whole wheat

• Olive oil, two tablespoons worth

• Basil that is fresh for garnishing

Directions

1. Ensure to heat the oven to 375 degrees Fahrenheit (190 degrees Celsius).

2. Apply olive oil to the eggplant slices, then bake them until they are soft.

3. A layer of marinara sauce, eggplant slices, mozzarella, and Parmesan cheese should be layered in a baking dish.

4. To finish, repeat the layers and sprinkle breadcrumbs on top. Bake until the mixture is bubbling and warm.

Nutritional Facts

• The number of calories is 350

15 grams of protein

Carbohydrates: thirty grams

10 grams of fiber

• 18 grams of healthy fats

Parfait of Cheesecake with Berry and Lemon

Ingredients

• Two fluid ounces of low-fat cream cheese

One-half cup of Greek yogurt

• One-fourth of a cup of honey

One lemon, with the zest and the juice

• One cup of a mixture of berries, including strawberries, blueberries, and raspberries

The crust calls for a half cup of almond meal.

Directions

1. Mix the cream cheese, Greek yogurt, honey, lemon zest, and lemon juice together in a bowl until the mixture is completely smooth.

2. Arrange the almond meal, cream cheese mixture, and mixed berries in a layering pattern in the serving glasses.

3. Continue to layer the ingredients, then finish with a berry topping.

Nutritional Facts

Total calories: 300

• Protein: ten grams

• 25 grams of carbohydrates

• Fiber content: 5 grams

• 18 grams of healthy fats

Tips:

Adapt the seasoning to your personal tastes in terms of flavor.

• To increase the nutritious content of your diet, consume lean proteins and entire grains.

• When presenting these dishes, take into consideration the nutritional requirements of each individual.

The purpose of these recipes for special occasions is to highlight the importance of renal health while simultaneously bringing joy to your joyful times. Not only are these recipes delicious, but they also contribute to general well-being because they are made with fresh ingredients and take into account the importance of maintaining a balanced diet. Take pleasure in these unique dishes with the people you care about while you create memories together at the table.

CHAPTER 9

Hints for the Planning and Preparation of Meals at Home

When it comes to leading a healthy lifestyle, meal planning and preparation are crucial components. These activities offer various advantages, including the opportunity to save time and money, as well as the capacity to make better-educated decisions regarding one's diet. These suggestions will assist you in streamlining the process of meal planning and preparation, regardless of whether you are concentrating on kidney health or just trying to improve your overall well-being.

1. Establish Realistic Objectives:

You should first determine your nutritional preferences and goals. Be honest with yourself about your ability to cook and the amount of time you have available to devote to the preparation of meals each week. To ensure that your meal planning is sustainable over the long term, it is important to set attainable goals.

2. Create a Menu for the Week

• Make a plan for your meals for the upcoming week. You should think about including a wide range of fruits, vegetables, whole grains, and proteins in your diet. In addition to ensuring that your meals are nutritionally balanced, a well-rounded menu also helps to keep your meals fascinating.

3. To Cook in Batches:

Large quantities of essential components, including grains, proteins, and vegetables, should be prepared in advance. Put these in the refrigerator or the freezer so that you can put them together quickly and easily on the weeknights. This reduces the amount of time you spend cooking each day and makes it easier for you to enjoy meals that you have prepared at home.

4. Discover The Latest Recipes:

Keep things interesting by experimenting with different recipes regularly. To meet your dietary requirements, you should look for dishes that are kidney-friendly. Experimenting with a wide range of flavors and cuisines not only provides variety to your meals but also helps you avoid being bored with your cooking.

5. Nutrient-rich foods Should Be Included:

• Make nutrient-dense foods that are beneficial to your overall health your first priority. Make sure that each of your meals has a variety of fruits and vegetables, lean meats, whole grains, and healthy fats throughout the rainbow. Ensure that the choices you make help to the health of your kidneys while also satisfying your overall dietary needs.

6. Mindful control of portion sizes:

• Pay attention to the sizes of the portions to prevent overeating. Plates and bowls of a smaller size can help control portion sizes. When it comes to maintaining a healthy balance, measurements of ingredients and keeping note of serving sizes can be of great assistance.

7. What to Do with Leftovers:

Ensure that you plan your meals with leftovers in mind. This results in less food being wasted and provides options that are convenient for meals or lunches in the future. To ensure that the quality of the leftover meals is preserved, it is important to keep them correctly.

8. Maintain a Pantry That Is Kidney-Friendly:

• Ensure that your cupboard is well-stocked with the essential foods that are kidney-proof. Things like broths with a low salt content, canned beans, whole grains, herbs, and spices are all examples of components that may be used in a wide variety of dishes.

9. Plan Days for Preparation:

• Set aside particular days a week for the preparation of meals. The preparation of vegetables, the marinating of proteins, or the cooking of grains in advance could all fall under this category. The cooking process is made more efficient throughout the hectic weekdays when the items that have been prepared are easily available.

10. Invest in Tools That Will Save You Time:

Consider investing in items for the kitchen that will save you time and effort. A slow cooker, an Instant Pot, or a food processor are examples of appliances that can dramatically cut down on the amount of time spent preparing meals by hand.

11. Maintain Your Hydration:

Include hydration as part of your meal planning process. To maintain healthy kidneys, water is necessary since it helps the kidneys eliminate waste products. Ensure that you are fulfilling the requirements for the amount of fluids you consume daily by keeping a water bottle on hand.

12. Take Care to Read the Labels:

In particular, pay strict attention to the information on food labels about the amount of sodium. When purchasing canned products and processed foods, go for ones that contain less sodium or no added salt. The monitoring of your sodium consumption is essential for maintaining healthy kidneys.

13. Talk things over with a dietitian:

If you have particular dietary limitations or concerns regarding your health, you might think about speaking with a trained dietician. They can provide individualized coaching, which will ensure that your meal planning is following your specific nutritional requirements.

14. Putting Mindfulness into Practice:

Eat slowly and relish each bite of your food. To cultivate the practice of mindful eating, pay attention to the flavors, textures, and how your body reacts to the food you are eating. Consequently, this may result in improved digestion as well as a deeper appreciation for the food you eat.

15. Prepare Snacks That Are Kidney-Friendly:

Make a plan and get ready some snacks that are safe for kidneys to have on hand. Snacks that are high in nutrients can offer additional nourishment in between meals and help prevent cravings for unhealthy foods. Take into consideration options such as fresh fruits, veggie sticks, or trail mix that has elements that are kidney-friendly.

16. Commemorate the Diversity:

It is important to consume a wide variety of foods to guarantee that you are getting a complete range of nutrients. Incorporate a wide variety of fruits, vegetables, proteins, and grains into your diet to celebrate the concept of diversity in your meals. This not only improves the nutritional value of meals but also makes them more fun to eat.

17. Make a plan for adaptability:

Maintain a flexible approach to your eating plan. Because of the unpredictability of life, it is not uncommon for plans to be altered. The ability to adapt to unforeseen circumstances while still making conscious decisions is made possible by having a flexible approach.

18. Maintain an Inventory of:

It is important to conduct regular inventory checks of your pantry, refrigerator, and freezer. Having a list of the components you already own allows you to avoid making purchases that aren't necessary and guarantees that you make use of the goods you already have before they go bad.

19. Put an end to burnout:

Simplifying your meal planning when necessary is an effective way to prevent burnout. When you are in a hurry, it is acceptable to consume meals that are simple and quick to prepare. Maintaining a sustainable approach to meal planning requires striking a balance between the convenience of the food and its nutritious content.

20. Delight in the Procedure:

Make the process of planning and preparing meals a part of your habit that you look forward to. Experiment with different flavors, involve members of your family, and take satisfaction in the fact that you are providing your body with nutritious meals that are kidney-friendly.

Through the implementation of these suggestions into your routine of meal planning and preparation, you will be able to cultivate a method that is both sustainable and pleasurable for nourishing your body while simultaneously supporting kidney health. Ensure that your meals are not just nutritious but also a source of pleasure and well-being by striking a balance between variety, nutrition, and convenience. This will ensure that your meals are delivered on all three fronts.

CHAPTER 10

Kidney-Friendly Meal Plan for the Next 7 Days

Beginning a journey to focus on kidney health for a period of 21 days requires careful meal planning to provide a balance of necessary nutrients while taking into consideration any dietary limitations that may be appropriate. This meal plan provides a selection of delectable foods that are suitable for kidneys, and they are included in the breakfast, lunch, supper, and snack categories. Remember to adjust the amount of your portions according to your unique requirements, and if you have any specific dietary problems, you should discuss them with a qualified medical practitioner.

Day one:

Smoothie with berries and lemon for breakfast

Quinoa salad with chickpeas and vegetables is what you'll find for lunch.

• Dinner will consist of steamed asparagus and baked salmon topped with a lemon-dill sauce.

The Greek yogurt with fresh berries is a delicious snack.

Day Two:

Avocado toast topped with tomato salsa is the breakfast option.

• Lunch: a soup made with lentils and vegetables

Served for dinner: grilled chicken breast, quinoa pilaf, and Brussels sprouts that have been roasted.

• Snack: a combination of seeds and nuts

Day 3:

Chia seed pudding with a variety of berries is served for breakfast.

The Spinach and Mushroom Omelette is the lunch option.

Brown rice and stuffed bell peppers with ground turkey make up the selection for dinner.

• Snack: Cucumber slices accompanied by hummus •

Day 4:

• A Greek yogurt parfait topped with granola and berries is served for breakfast.

• Wrap made with whole wheat, stuffed with turkey, avocado, and spinach for lunch

Dinner will consist of a mixed green salad and eggplant parmesan.

A snack consisting of fresh watermelon slices

Day 5:

Oatmeal with sliced bananas and almond butter is what you'll find for breakfast.

Quinoa and black bean bowl with roasted vegetables is what you'll find for lunch.

The dinner menu consists of baked cod with a lemon-herb crust and quinoa salad.

A snack consisting of Edamame Pods seasoned with a pinch of sea salt

Day 6:

Breakfast consists of a bowl of mixed berry smoothies.

A Greek salad topped with grilled chicken is for lunch.

• An evening meal consisting of stir-fried tofu, broccoli, and brown rice

• A snack consisting of cottage cheese topped with pineapple salsa

Day 7:

• For breakfast, we have pancakes made with whole grains and fresh berries.

Lentil and vegetable stir-fry to be served for lunch

Meatballs made with turkey, served with zucchini noodles and marinara sauce for dinner

The trail mix with nuts and dried cranberries is a great snack option.

Day 8:

• For breakfast, scrambled eggs topped with feta cheese and spinach

• For lunch, we make stuffed peppers with quinoa and vegetables.

Grilled shrimp skewers and lemon-herb quinoa are available for dinner.

Served as a snack, apple slices topped with almond butter

Day 9:

For breakfast, we recommend the Kidney-Friendly Recipe for Banana Walnut Muffins.

The Caprese Salad with Balsamic Glaze is the lunch option.

Dinner consists of chicken and vegetable kebabs served over couscous.

Carrot sticks dipped in hummus; this is a snack.

Day 10:

Breakfast: a smoothie made with blueberries and almonds

Spinach and feta cheese stuffed chicken breasts are the lunch option.

Cooked lentil curry served over brown rice for dinner

Cottage cheese and cherry tomatoes make for a delicious snack.

The kidney-friendly meal plan that is included in this 7-day plan offers a wide variety of recipes that will keep your meals interesting while also promoting the best possible kidney health. Following your individual preferences, you are free to repeat your favorite recipes or substitute items. It is important to remember to drink plenty of water and to make adjustments to meet your specific dietary requirements. When it comes to fostering a lifestyle that is kidney-friendly and sustainable, consistency is essential.

When you nourish your kidneys, you nourish your life for the rest of your life.

CONCLUSION

You are making a substantial investment in your overall well-being by beginning a path to prioritize kidney health through the implementation of a diet that is kidney-friendly and comes with careful planning. With this 21-day meal plan, you will have access to a thoughtful and varied collection of meals that have been developed to provide care for your kidneys while also satisfying your taste buds. Now that we have reached the end of this guide, let us take a moment to contemplate the fundamental concepts and the influence they can have on your lifestyle and health.

Striking a Balance:

To achieve and maintain kidney health, it is necessary to strike a careful balance in the choices that you make regarding your food. The meal plan emphasizes the significance of ingesting a wide range of foods that are rich in nutrients, such as fruits, vegetables, lean proteins, and whole grains. The maintenance of this equilibrium ensures that you will acquire the necessary vitamins and minerals while also preserving the health of your kidneys.

The Health Advantages of Mindful Eating:

Eating mindfully involves not only the food that you consume but also how you consume it. Spending time to appreciate and enjoy each meal not only improves the overall quality of your eating experience but also helps your digestive system function more efficiently. By taking this method, you will be able to cultivate a more positive connection with food, where you will be able to appreciate the sustenance that it offers.

Versatile and long-term sustainable:

The 7-day meal plan is devised to be flexible enough to accommodate your individual preferences and requirements. It is quite acceptable to substitute items, to repeat recipes that you enjoy, or to adjust the serving sizes following your specific needs. The objective is to develop a method of nourishing your body that is both sustainable and pleasurable, to promote not only renal health but also a more comprehensive lifestyle.

Teaching and empowering individuals:

Knowledge is a powerful tool, and having an awareness of the impact that your dietary choices have on the health of your kidneys gives you the ability to make decisions that are informed. The dishes that are included in this meal plan have been developed with this information in mind. They not only provide scrumptious meals, but they also serve as a basis for making decisions that are more health-conscious after the 7 days have passed.

Personalized Consultation and Alterations:

However, even though this book offers a thorough meal plan, it is essential to acknowledge the fact that the health profile of each individual is different. If you have special dietary issues or medical conditions, you should think about speaking with a qualified dietitian or a healthcare expert. They can provide individualized coaching to ensure that the meals you choose are in perfect alignment with the health goals you have set for yourself.

A Trip as Opposed to a Final Destination:

Making kidney health a priority is not a task that can be completed quickly; rather, it is a journey. A kickstart, the 7-day meal plan is a means to integrate healthy behaviors into your daily life. They are a way to get you started. The more you proceed, the more likely it is that you will come across new recipes, modify your preferences, and figure out what works best for you. Honor even the most insignificant of your accomplishments, maintain your dedication, and welcome the road toward long-term renal health.

To summarize, providing proper nourishment to your kidneys is not solely dependent on the foods that you consume; rather, it is about adopting a way of life that promotes your overall health and wellness. You are not only improving the health of your kidneys by practicing mindful eating, making well-informed decisions, and committing to a diet that is better for your kidneys, but you are also laying the groundwork for a life that is healthier and more full of vitality. I raise a glass to your journey toward nourishing yourself, achieving wellness, and ensuring that your kidneys become healthier.